STROLLING DOWN HEAVEN'S GATE

Gisele B. Vincent-Page

Strolling Down Heaven's Gate

Strolling Down
Heaven's Gate

Gisele B. Vincent-Page

authorHOUSE®

AuthorHouse™
1663 Liberty Drive
Bloomington, IN 47403
www.authorhouse.com
Phone: 1-800-839-8640

First published by AuthorHouse   08/12/2011

ISBN: 978-1-4634-3729-9 (sc)
ISBN: 978-1-4634-3728-2 (ebk)

Library of Congress Control Number: 2011912749

Printed in the United States of America

Any people depicted in stock imagery provided by Thinkstock are models, and such images are being used for illustrative purposes only.
Certain stock imagery © Thinkstock.

This book is printed on acid-free paper.

.....dedicated to Joelle, Yves, Guy, Amber

I would like to acknowledge the beautiful and generous use of Diane Isaac, Walter Isaac and Garry Robinson's photography.

Contents

SUCH GIFTS

I've been listening to the trees all my life.
Fifty years later, I understand they have
been talking to me.
Whispering, willowing waves of branches
and leaves. Saying we love you. We are the
tickle in your ears, whispering words of peace.
Soothing your eyes in times of grief.

Sing to the joy of emptiness, we smooth away
your fears; we bathe you in the grace of giving.

Giving is the greatest gift.
Giving away your name, your ego, your shame.
Giving you forgiveness. Give what you have
learnt. Knowledge is a sharing gift. How can it
be a secret?

The wind is heavenly music.

Exhausted Numb

This is the state I arrived in at the Palliative Care Ward at Riverview Hospital in March, 2010. I remained there till June. There was no imminent danger of death. Just a confusion and exhaustion. Sitting at home with a dog who was driving me nuts, staring at walls and windows that drove me insane. A stomach that would not function. It held on to everything I ingested and the myriad of substances that I took to make "me go" didn't do much for my mental and physical constitution. I was a wonderful patient. "Gisele is self-directed" the nurse would tell her students who tagged along with her and they would marvel. They spent what seemed like hours taking notes about everything. I babbled about Buddha and meditation. I should have kept my mouth shut. I was much too entertaining. I should have stayed in my pyjamas. I looked much too good. I showered every day. I should have left some stink on me. "Well, if you need anything, you know who to call," they would say walking out the door. By the end of winter I could only grit my teeth.

I had friends who called. I had friends who didn't call. Very few knew what to say, no matter how much I coached them. Visiting times were set up so I wouldn't tire too much. My kids did groceries for me or I ordered them from the store. I did the laundry. There was a cleaning lady sent every two weeks to clean and do laundry, but by the time I had prepared the house for her arrival, I was exhausted.

They weren't allowed to touch or move anything, so the vacuuming and the dusting was pretty scant. I'd have to keep the dog in her kennel and we'd close the door to my painting room where I blew my cigarette smoke out the window; just like I used to do when I was a kid. Sometimes a cleaning person would show up unannounced and I'd be so bamboozled I'd send them away.

My brain felt like it was degenerating.

One day, the nurse didn't know what to do with me. I couldn't talk; I had nothing to say. She said I seemed very angry. What a surprise, sitting at home for over a year having been pronounced "dying" and not knowing what I was supposed to do. She asked if maybe I'd like to go to the hospital; like we were going for ice-cream or something. She phoned my brother to inform him and the whole family was set in turmoil.

Time

Wish I had worn a watch so I would
know the time of day.
But does it really matter anyway.

Time comes and goes, watch the sun,
it will help you find your way.

You can plan your day away
or
let the plan make your day.

Either way you make it to the
moonfall
whether your watch is on
or
just on for display.

God's Face

The colours that billow
underneath those pillows
that you hug
are really the fellows
that sing and dance
readying you
and your new
space, that now you
can really face.

Beautiful beings knocking at the core
that is no longer sore.
Smoothness and ease are all you're really
waiting for. In a blink of an eye
you'll be taken to the core.

This journey is for the beauty that stands
at your door.
Just knock and come in.
There, might be the portal.

The birds will sing as they did before,
the bells will ring
pealing all the lives you've
gone through before.

80'S Aids Anxiety

I was there in the early 1980's when AIDS ruled like a demon on a planet gone mad with fear; with masks, gowns and gloves; with warning signs posted on hospital doors: ISOLATION. I was saturated with fear and folly. I stumbled and tripped all over myself; skirting around this and that; vague in responses to questions about what was wrong with John, my husband lying in the Intensive Care Unit. The truth was too horrible to repeat. We told our parents vague stories of sexual experimentation and told our children that it was a private family matter. I behaved like a crazy person. I refused to be tested at the time. I couldn't risk the reality of more bad news. Whatever I did do, I was preserving myself and my family. I had no roadmaps, no indicators, hints or cues on how to behave or react . . .

There was a lack of imagination in the 1980's; despite the great boon of sexual freedom. We had no words or language to adequately explain what was happening to us. Words like isolation and contagion took root. Our thoughts, our feelings ran rampant with negative possibilities. The spectrum of sexual expression between men and women; men and men; women and women weren't accessible in our conversations back then.

A stigma plastered a whole community of people, isolating them from the rest of the world. Judgement camps were formed: the good, the bad, the innocent and the guilty.

Fears left no room for thoughts of love and relationships. Silent judgements reigned. I chose silence; drove myself into isolation. Anxiety was paramount. We were protecting ourselves from . . . the unknown.

. . . . at Riverview, my spirits improved, but my mobility degenerated as I had plenty of space to walk and walk I did till . . .

Angels On High

There are angels that walk this sight.
Hands outstretched ready to catch
flight. Face of sweetness arms so strong.

Please sir, help me before I fall
arm in arm we walked the spread
to the door, I'm Gisele, I'm from
the third floor; I'm from the fourth;
I visit my wife. Steady and sturdy,
he didn't let go. His arm led my
whole body to the door of safety
and sureness.

Thank you, how can I thank you
for your lack of hesitation for
breaking my fall. My angel on call.

From The Mall To The River

Do you know how much energy it took for you to play?
Just sit here. Just be.

You've whirled and twirled like a spinning top
just let the breeze ease your grasp, your gaze
at what is past.
Like the river flowing its natural path
this time of holding him closely was the best.

Gently, gently you must breathe and don't let
your big feet get in the way; your arms and
legs carry you astray.

Go smoothly down each path follow the sun, go
quietly down each way. Our time together, alone here in
May. You've run all my errands
held me at each curb, each blade of grass.

You're big and strong but inside your heart is
breaking. I promise you I'll always be here
and in dying, I won't be in pain.
When we meet again, we'll keep the
pace slow; we'll keep that urgency
in your gait back down to its sacred place.

Solace

Surrounded by my angels of care
who have seen me in my underwear wiped away my tears
of pain.

Soothed my burning feet in ice;
changed my dressings, shook
their heads at what they see
burning sore that just shouldn't be.

They shelter you from these gruesome sights so we can
just BE here in delight.

. . . Hiv . . . Lives . . . Here . . .

I have lived with HIV for twenty-seven years. HIV is a pronouncement, a judgement of one's life. It is a disease like cancer, Parkinson's, multiple sclerosis and many other long-term chronic and debilitating diseases that exist in today's world. However, unlike other diseases, HIV still carries a stigma. What are your expectations of a person with HIV? Would it be your child's teacher? Your sister, your cousin, your co-worker? An IV drug-user; a prostitute? It's often difficult to determine who lives with HIV. For 27 years, my life has been a twisting and turning of events as I learnt to put on the right face, the required persona. Was it mother, friend, daughter, sister, or teacher? Fortunately, I had a degree in Dramatic Studies and those skills came in handy as I weaved my way through the daily doings of being a widowed mother of three children.

Who would you tell? Your parents? Which of your friends? How would you explain the ISOLATION signs on your husband's hospital door? Or why all the medical staff and visitors wore masks, gowns and gloves? Many of us say nothing. This silence only increases the stigma.

Today, I like to think I'm in a safer place, closer to death than to life, having let go of the side-stepping of the truth; of having raised three children to productive adulthood; being rid of many obligations as I float in palliative care which is both a wall of safety and nuisance. Is it safe, even now, after 27 years to speak freely of what is ordinary to me but still completely foreign and skewed to the masses? Now that I am no longer looking into the abyss; what role did HIV play in my life?

GOD TOUCHES ME

My shoulders are blades of flesh
They hold my skinny arms
To hands that hold this pen
across this page as it reaches
the end of a long lived life that was
meant to bend fold and remend.

But these feet have already
left; I can feel it in my chest.
These lips want to smile the
day away; I have nothing elsc to say.

Knees to my chin how long has that been;
to crouch, cuddle what is now so
thin. Press and pull, it all fits in.

The warmth and the cool these toes are not mine,
they belong to the sublime. Up my pants you will find
my legs weak and spindly. A jelly belly that shakes in my
tummy; my thin arms hold loops of skin. They are faraway
and my head needs covering but the sun warms it and my
face is full of laughter
because God has reached out his hand to me.

Rainbows And Angels

Wakeful profound relaxing, let go into life as it is.
Happiness is already here. Pieces of paper ribbons
and bow; colors on paper I love you.

Ribbons in her hair chocolates to share, simple
truths from a small simple being reaches through
the crusts of years.
One look, one glance and the crusts disappear.

Open your eyes, see with your ears the beautiful
rays of sunshine a child holds within.
Fleeing hair dust in the wind sparkles on her fingers,
chocolate milk within, surrender to this infinite awareness
search for God within.

Setting sun living air, a spirit impels and rolls through all
things, meet into the sun; just having fun. May I be at
peace in the small holdings of a little child's hand, a hug so
sublime taking you to other lands, where teddy bears rule.

I am with you be praised with this great humility.
The beauty of children's faces peering at you,
sticky golden fingers, just having fun.
One ribbon tying the other one undone.

Heart melts to pieces, once glued and glum,
your past now your present is also having
all the fun.

You too can be this powerful imp of fun,
sunshine emotion simplicity wilfulness
unspeakable curiosity.

Simple steps, acts of love in a line drawing
innocent and giving sharing unparalleled
expecting nothing but love. You give
easily. What's to hold behind like a fountain
that keeps spinning. You sit and like this
learning from this little holder of the sun;
dancing her dervish dance playing you into
a trance of love building upon love building.

God, am I looking for you? I am with my
little urchin showing me the way to forgotten
places, traces of how it was to play in
gardens from far away.

This is where I want to stay.

DEALS AND BARGAINS

I made deals with God. The biggest bargain: raising my children to adulthood.

PLAN A: I would leave them in the care of family members. My secret plan was to greet my eldest daughter's grade 12 graduation and 18th birthday. I knew, despite the enormous sacrifice I was imposing on her, that she would look after her two younger brothers. These two milestones were celebrated with the traditional cakes and candles; family gathered and happy birthdays and congratulations were proclaimed. Meanwhile I harboured a quiet secret song of success in my heart: this wish, this bargain achieved. When my second child, my son reached his age of adulthood and graduation; I had another double celebration: the public and the private thanksgiving for one less worry. He too, would accept responsibility for the rearing of his younger brother. If I were to die then, the baby of the family would continue to live with familiar faces with no need to dismantle his life and him off to relatives. Just a few more years till the "baby" now an adolescent, would attain his own adulthood . . . and when he did, I looked around during the graduation ceremony for signs of recognition of the monumental event that was occurring in my heart. Fruitions of events that were completely out of my hands were finished. No matter that the church was appallingly hot in our June heat packed with hundreds of family members applauding their young graduates; it didn't matter that I was alone with this achievement. I had arrived somewhere safe and spacious. I could breathe easier; dying became easier to face. I can't recapture the states of fear and anxiety that I lived through the simplest daily activities. I look back with curiosity and shake my head in recognition of what I let fear do to me.

At the palliative care ward, I turned inward for strength. So many of MY needs were met. My meals, my bed, my laundry. Strangely, I felt I had control of my living. My needs to talk, to explain; to converse about what was happening to me and my family. Here, my nerves were smoothed, the right questions were asked. I felt protected. I wasn't being diverted and placated. I could use my time to find beautiful places, to grow, to meet new people, to offer support, to be useful. To reflect, to pray and even smile.

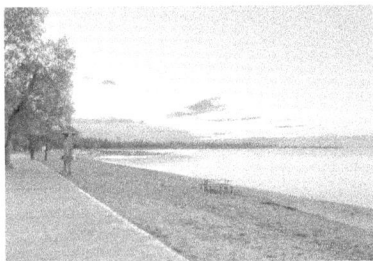

A Simple Day

Did you ever have a day where
everything went your way?
From last minute hair appointments
and deliveries made just as you were
about to give way?

When people bring you gifts that far
exceeded anything you ever expected?

Did you? Did you?

A day where your favourite bench in
the sun opens up as you glide by
hoping it is free?

And it is! And it is!

Did you ever have such a day
where everything is going your
way?

Well, I have! I have! I have!

KNOWLEDGE . . . WISDOM

I had many opportunities to teach. I had many classrooms and students. I taught many subjects in both French and English. I wandered through numerous topics and HEALTH was one of them. My classrooms were my refuge.

These realms I filled with laminated pictures of Picasso, Van Gogh and numerous other impressionists. They played right beside the French verbs and English novels. This was my queendom. I reigned there. My walls to adorn, my desks to straighten and a wealth of books to play in. And of course, my kids, the students. My solace of safety untouched by AIDS. Or was it?

I taught many classes about HIV as required by the school curriculum. I certainly never spoke about me and my AIDS. Where was my story in those lessons? Just how much did I deprive my students of the truth; of any real knowledge? So, AIDS did find its way into my royal realm of safety.

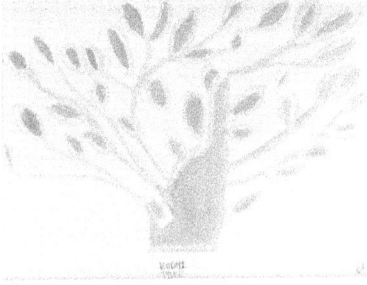

CHARACTERS

You probably don't remember me, you and a dog named Boo?
Well this was more like Clifford, Daryl and Tic Tac Tom;
from Winnipeg, Rankin Inlet and Aberdeen. Three more
unlikely characters couldn't possibly be.
Friends forever. This is how it came to be.
They were damaged by stroke, of the heart
that left them immobile and damaged.
I was on the sidelines; put on hold in a
holding place called Palliative Care.
The smoke shack drew us together
with me painting the Bodhi Tree.
Exchanging stories that exacted honesty.
Tales of fishing in the sea, of friends robbing
you blind, even Daryl's TV. Shared tales of
illness, work in progress and a God that we
all could see. Limbs and hearts moved me to
tears till even I shared the pains of my soul.
Then one day we clasped each other's hands
to our hearts. Power and strength flowed through
me. Heaven sent the hand that wiped the tear from
my cheek.
This is how the unlikely meeting came to be, Tom
Tic Tac, Daryl, Clifford and me.

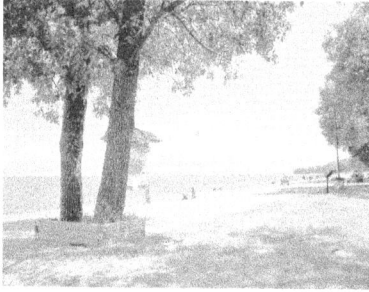

WATER

WAVES

Great waves on the stones giving me space to
absorb the grace of my life, so rich.

I can hardly believe that this great beauty is in store for
me. Hard clean water slapping the shore has opened the
door to the place I am meant for

I was scared and I screamed my body bent in
two ; God's power squeezed me and tore at my soul;
strength went out of control.

Like a fool, I thought I was ready.
I was scared for my eyes, my hands and my legs at the gate
slapping the shore. Calling me in and I

was afraid of closing the door to
infinite goodbyes
and new plans for those staying
at the shore.

Goodbye my children, my family, my friends.

Having found the end of my journey
at the lake's edge. The Beloved takes
your hands and shows you the way.
There should be nothing to fear at this
fruitful end. Elements are harsh and
steady,

knowing when it is the breath's end.

Slowly, slowly, we will merge with
the vast edge of the cosmic water
from whence we have been.

Return, return, to this endless line
just at the turn of the bend.

RAW

I am struck raw with this bleeding
heart; drips, dropping, straining
the pores of so many open sores

needles pricked in one more.
I am struck raw, wretched, stabbed
and torn; old bleeding sores
left dripping by the door.

We won't leave this way but
you already have many times
before.

. . . . MORE WATER

I hear water, waves upon waves of water. But I'm sitting here in snowy Winnipeg. No matter, my mind is on the beach; on all beaches I've spent days just sitting by the lapping waves, napping . . . resting my eyes . . . Hoarding images for a day just like today, when I would not be there. My eyes seized shut to replay for this day, a snowy day in Winnipeg. The children play and laugh in the distance; splashy sounds; droplets at my feet. That's where HIV lived, in the back of my mind, constant like a rock. A reminder of my brief stay on this earth.

BEACHES

Today, I do yearn for things of the past; for the warm wind on my skin and the sand between my toes; of somnolence by the shore; baskets of beach toys and Kool-Aid. The simplicity of spending the day at the beach. The sand scraping my feet. I was there too. The children laid on their towels sunning their backs; threw their bodies in the waves bringing them back. Too far, too far I say! They wave and just keep swimming away. HIV was there too, enjoying the day.

These water dreams made me yearn and an overnight stay at my brother's cottage was arranged. A beautiful place where I had spent many summers. My daughter and my son accompanied me, the nurses packed and arranged for all my medications. We drove down the highway with Stevie Wonder blasting on high.

No, the sun didn't show its face, but the rain and wind blew steadily. My son took care of all the fires, indoors and out. I sat cozily on the couch, having my feet massaged till I could feel them circulate again and I was tucked into bed. The next day, my daughter agreed to my dogged desire to be by the water and the waves bored into my soul.

Angel With An Umbrella

Encumbered with the walker
blankets for the wet bench,
sheets of water splashing the cement.
I ventured to my smoking spot
face hidden inside my hooded coat

I light my fire stick,

letting drops of water
reverberate on my hood.

My angel came walking by
called my name;

gave me her umbrella and kept on walking.

TEARS

Tears in the hallway
Tears in the bedroom
Tears in the I kitchen
Tears in the common room

Tears in my throat

Great heaving sobs of pain and sorrow.
There is no tomorrow
Who lets this be?
This place of grief and sorrow,
what does it matter, cry
cry like there's no tomorrow.

Tears come from the Beloved.
She knows your sorrow
crying lets hearts bleed,
letting out the sorrow.

The dying are sorry for
this heaping hollow.
The place where the
Beloved holds your sorrow.

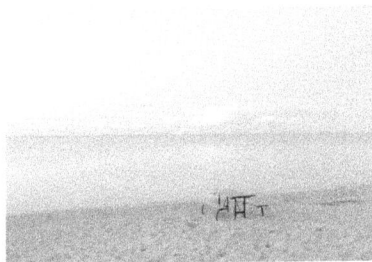

Bathing In The Rain

Droplets of rain are beautiful
they smooth away the pain.
A soft sheen, smoothed skin.
We bathe together
on this plain-edged
tree releasing the fragrance
and the pain.

For who are we but droplets of rain?

REMISSION

When I developed ocular shingles, I wore a patch, but it proved to be too little, too late. The virus and the bacteria had long taken the vision in my left eye With great anger, I researched and questioned. I obsessed evenings on the internet. Disappointment grew as it appeared to me that certain simple measures had not been taken to specifically protect the cornea from bacterial infection. I stewed and brooded like a baby at this injustice. One day a student approached me and pointed out that we used, "to laugh" in this class, have fun and joke around . . . what's wrong?" Her face was full of question and bewilderment. I ended my search to find a culprit. I put all my files of paper and websites of "proof" that a wrong had been done into a large manila envelope in the back of a drawer. I resolved to end this pain I was creating for myself and now for others; my innocent students. What was I teaching them? What was I learning? We would laugh again in this classroom. AIDS would not have control here in my "queendom". I would continue to search the path of real schooling: wisdom. However, being a long-term survivor is not an event for celebration. It is still just more pronouncement. I am judged. Who celebrates the long-timers? Who says, "Hurrah", good for you. You made it! The energy it takes to survive is monumental. With HIV, it's just endurance. It is not a celebration; merely perplexing. There's no recognition of achievement; just more of the same sad music. The threatening undertones of uncertainty simmer non-stop. Having lived this way for 27 years, I've come to realize, despite the wonderful family and friends I have had, that this life with HIV is a burden. There is no real remission with HIV, just an infection, bacterial or viral, and we recover, time and again, leaving our bodies weaker and weaker. Our sickness wails in silence, the song of rejoicing is small and inaudible. Our language is still weak and unsatisfactory. We continue to be judged. One day, in the early summer of 2010, I was sitting in the smoke shack of the Palliative Care facility when a very fine woman who had suffered a lot with cancer, asked me quite respectfully, if she could inquire as to the ailment that brought us together. I replied, "HIV", which I've had for 26 years. She nodded her head in empathy but her words, though spoken with kindness were: I don't judge you." She meant well, but if I had said "cancer", would the word "judge" have any reason to come up?

HEAVEN'S GATE

With so many gifts to
surrender
I can't empty myself fast enough
so much to give so much to
live, the finishing line is
clear
and clearer every minute
every second I breathe.
It's time to go
release
reform refit relax
refill repent
relieve
relive in small bits
the soft smells and gentle hits.
Agree and be with the flow of
emptiness
let it flow enjoy the newness of
saying goodbye in slow waves
lapping in your soul.
A soft sea, like an ocean that slows at the
ridge of your feet. Be rich and glow with
light that calls you home. Lilacs still bloom,
you feed what you don't eat to the great sea
of gentility.

Just Another Storm

This wind like so many winds is not going
to chase me away
I'll bind myself like a rock
weather just like every other storm
that's come my way.

Why would I collapse in this one?
I'll anchor myself to the Beloved,
rid myself of this fear and vulnerability.
Grasp the compassionate One. Look
into the eyes of unconditional love.
See the faces of my mother, of John,
of my father, my brother, of Buddha
or the almighty God.

Experience this compassionate being
wanting to be here with me; hold on
to this merciful presence. The sun
peeks in and out, leaving space to
envelop and stir me from my slumber.

A hand reaches out and covers mine
I'm here I'm here we're all here.

Let go and forgive yourself for being human.

WHERE WHAT WHEN

Life is a circle. I was sitting outside the palliative care ward where I resided till I could be "placed". I observed the winding road I used to travel daily to and from the school I taught at for five years. It is also the same road I used to walk my border collie Sheba. I knew this bend of road because I had lived near it too; in a huge house I bought shortly after John died. The river, the trees, the bend and the cars, the people who traffic it don't seem to have changed a bit. Today, I don't think I've changed a bit either. I've continued to experience both good and awful experiences with HIV. When I had occasion to speak to medical students about LIVING WITH A TERMINAL ILLNESS; I received beautiful cards of gratitude and praise. One student wrote a beautiful BA'HAI prayer for me. Such moments of kindness are easy to treasure. No sooner does the beauty of these moments simmer in my soul does a fresh eye-opening event come to slap me in the face with the other side of reality. Like the shame I experienced when I was rejected from a care home because I had HIV. I know the shame is not really mine to bear, but I was treated shamefully. That's when the abyss opens up again? What to do? Where to go?

INFINITY

Fear of infinity sits with me
today, eternity flies, looms,
hovers, stretches the heart
must make room for the
dark

space I am to embark.
Though I let my eyes search
for God within;
let my eyes mingle with
the Cosmic wind.

Afraid of what will be
stormy slaps. It is not
really your place to
see such a grace as this.

The thorny drift burnished
by that crush around the
trees. Now I'm afraid God,
now I'm glad you are here with me.

WORDS

Farewell to another soul
bless you, I love you
I think of you
I am on a new path.

Which one? What kind?
Does it matter? Need it be
named? Another me is
growing out tenderly

needing to be cropped and cuddled
rocked to sleep a new me,
whose legs can't be trusted
to keep the old beat

faces, are they looking at me?

The time on any watch is wrong.

Smoking And Reflecting

I had occasion to reflect, to look inside, to spend time with Walter, who helped me center myself again. I prayed. I meditated. I chanted. Every morning I would rise early, make or buy a coffee; I wore a jacket with many pockets; one tucked with my digital recorder on which I had recorded reflections, prayers and meditations. In another pocket, I tucked in my CD player so I could listen and chant with GRACE. I would sign myself out at the front desk and make my way down three floors, by elevator and walk a fairly long bit of sidewalk to the smoking shack. Because it was early spring, it was cold and sometimes it rained. Smoking staffers would come and go, weaving themselves in and out of my prayers. I grew to see that they were my prayers, as they shared their family and work news, joked and laughed. We often watched the sunrise over the river. That was my favourite way to start the day.

One day walking back from the shack, with the sun now at my back, the idea opened up in my brain and in my heart: I wanted to be by the WATER! I knew there was a senior's complex at Winnipeg Beach and with the help of my social worker and a myriad of assistants, we began the process of applications and paperwork . . . sunrises, water, sand, sunsets . . . that's where I belonged.

Fullness Of Freedom

Then the sun came out
liberation from the cold and wet.

I hope you're a good cook as I
set the hospital tray before her.
Laughter leaves the room with
stories of failed lemon meringue
pies. Events moving backwards
and forwards. I've never known
such emptiness; non-attachment.

My soul yells live on, make a list
of things to do. The sun will be
out. I'm out of breath. So excited
about your life; now that you've
walked into my death. I'll have
coffee for my friends; more
paintings for their eyes. I have
gifts and time to share, I welcome
phone calls that agree with my
serenity. Free to give what no
longer belongs to me you see
what I cherish.

LIFE AT WINNIPEG BEACH
THE GIFT OF WIND

winding scarves on my face
blowing air through my skin
skirting around my legs searching
in my soul rooting out the pegs
of memory of other winds of
time spaceless nameless
places and scenes that are
past and gone lifted up out of
sorrow far away gone gone
long gone free with the wind

CHANGE

Leg to the left or is it to the right
call this change. I do not need to remember
that most of all, it's no big
deal. Just keep moving, one
way or the other.

God is on this path too,
he won't forsake you.

Eat with your mouth open
or is it close it when you chew?
It is all quite irrelevant in the end
what you decide to do. All doors
open. Pick one, if you must. They
are a little sticky, stuck in the muck

or slicky, shiny, free from dust.
Each of them exactly where you should
be. Slippery, stuck shiny or gooey, there
is no need to feel gloomy. They will all
feel the same.

There's no shame in seeking out God's world
in his name. It has been left for us,
let us bring fame, pain,or glory in the
Beloved's name.

WARMTH

I sit in the sun and take it all in,
arrive to meet the light that has
been living within each particle
of my sight.

Blind I have been to keep it all in,
move with the wind hear its calling.
It's faraway din. Don't be polite,
don't walk around me, come closer
so I can feel you within.

Tree Of Time

Liberty released by this seventy year
old tree bark mellowed burrowed
with eternity.

What is time doing here
no punch clock time clock
taking off my socks remind

God of my feet
don't forget these
sandboxed in serenity shade
from calm leaves awash
with rays; sweetness,

Synchronized swimmers follow
the sun pulled by no one no
thing; but having fun.

God's Rays

I like this body hot
from the rays God
blends.
All souls in their
proper spot.

stewed simmered steamed
colors orange yellow baby blue
which one are you? flip flops
thongs shades and hues
picnics and ice-cream too
umbrellas towels made only for
this grand sacred sand land.

GOD'S BREW

Is it hot or is it hot? Did I puke or did I puke?
First, it was peculiar before supper,
but at noon, it was hot and we sat
on the boardwalk.
Drank slurpees; ate frozen yogurt
cranberry and raspberry yum.
That was after lunch at Bonnie's
a breakfast place that closes at
three opens at six am
but only serves bacon and ham
till eleven lunch all around caesar salad
a quarter pound of croutons
shoved to the rim, dressing nice and garlicky.
It was the last thing that
catapulted itself from my
tummy
long after emitting dinner
of salad fish and tea.
A night to remember
barf bowls and bed changes
but it was clear by two am
that it was food poisoning
and not the flu or god knows what other
concoction god could brew.

A New Day

I hear you whittling, whistling and cawing.
Bird songs waking us. Come on, get up and
play.

caw caw away

You make me smile, my head is dizzy with
what will I do today.
Walk, dear God. Thank you.
I have my legs, these arms, these hands
keep this pen moving. I have a lot to say.

These tree-surrounded benches are my mainstay;
which one shall I choose for a sit and a stay?
A chat or a nod might be all I have to say,
thank you for the grace of a brand new day.

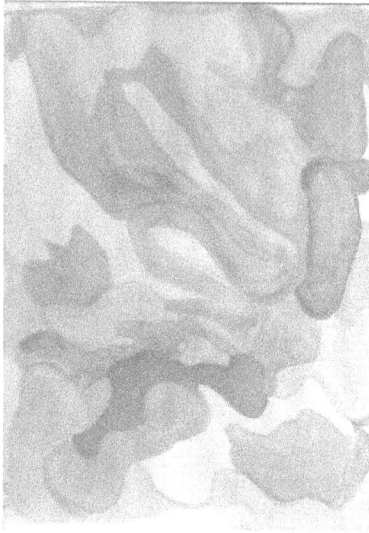

THE DIVINE MOOD

The divine mood visited me
today. Sitting by the water
tearing my heart away.

As worlds fell into parts,
my being, my breath
fell apart, exhale.
Breathe out. Make
room for the Divine Heart.

Warm and toasty a warm cinnamon bun
like a cat, sleep in the sun. There is so little
warmth; eyes have a hard time
focusing; the best part of the day is done.
Five am prayers; six am e-mails.

45

Beautiful walk in the sun
coffee and the fish fly gallery.
Tiredness reaches my soul.
There is a hole where there
was none.
A space is opening and thy will
be done. What to do with this
fatigue; we rest here or there
but I am in the sun with the Beloved.

LAST VISIT

Sitting in the sun
me, you, baby, nephew and brother too.
sand toys water ice cream blue

no longer one with nature my whole
body went numb.

Talk of past angers when our times
weren't fun
you read my mind completely
had not seen each other since
1991.

Hugging kissing think of you too!
If this was our last meeting, so be it

my well of silence just deepened a
little bit

SITTING

It is easy to love when all
you love sits with you, ripples
of water rolling, a stream, a trickle
flowing every square.

Try to be fair, you do have to
share this glory by the water
in the calm warm night air.

I found a shortcut
straight to the beach
right across the grass,
no detours upswing
or down. Just a straight
walk through this small
town.

My well of silence grows
brighter with each passing
hour.

Screaming kids should stay
away
when I want to pine
away. Sway with the water
as slowly as my breath may.

Poor Dying Me

The sun shines way too much,
pulsates this drug-filled body
I know that much.

Preserving heat in memory of those colder
days huddled in a smoking shack; where
else to stay dry and smoke my days away?

All right all right
I'll move
to a shade spot maybe
make myself another day
with my son who surprised
me with a visit today
bearing gifts of home grown
lettuce, much coveted tofu
senna tea, a credit card which
helps me deal with my sprees
relieves the burden of weekend
plan-making for his brother's trip to me.

We both know his sister is angry, as
she is entitled to be.

Shade spots keep my brain from churning the
methadone the wrong way, my white arabian
scarf keeps the sun's rays at bay.

Inhale

A break with the dead
between one and two p.m.
my breath labours a bit
skips beats

With every small kick of
a pebble or
a stone

Doors open wide or small
I float to another zone.
Exhale

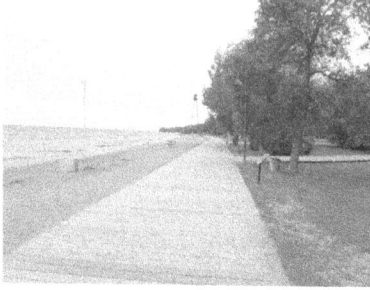

STROLLING SOULS

I swore I would quit writing on bits of paper
that's what a computer is for.

But how could I know that on day,
at four-forty in the afternoon of a
post-fair Monday, that I would
finally realize what I was here for.

I must have been drunk on something
when I arrived but now this is truly alive.

In the well of my soul, I must have opened the wrong
door looking for my sanity . . . I just spun frantically,
exhausting myself all the more.

Tranquility itself has just breezed through the core
of my dying; body quite like nothing before.

The tour shows, the bandstands and hellos; how do you dos.

Dangling earrings interfered with the score of music which

rolls from the shore, birds chirp so loudly how could I ignore

the message of love, safety, promising more heavenly
surprises, sunsets, sands and stones.

I'm not here to ignore the pain of others
so much room;

expand grow love don't huddle
time to cuddle.

Beach Bag Block

Let this be the last vision I see
boardwalk sand lake
bathing suits too tight
too droopy.

Stillness of sand, though at places
bumpy; the search for the right
spot. Blankets, chairs tucked
under bags of food and languages
foreign; they all say: the sand is hot,
the water is cold; I'll take this, you
take that.

Sunscreen and sunhat
no wonder I can't sleep
I get so anxious
to get right back
here to
this spot.

God made beaches so he can reach us.
If you don't see God's work here,
you'll need more than suntan lotion
for protection from this projection
of
perfection.

HIV is really just another element of our human imperfection. It's not a punishment, any more than cancer is a punishment. I once heard a preacher say to the congregation gathered in the chapel of the Palliative Care Ward, that: "death was a punishment for our sins". I wondered just how comforting that was to the small group of dying patients who had come to hear words of solace and comfort; at least, that was why I went.

My favourite experience with HIV occurred ar Riverview Hospital, where an elderly man of approximately 70 years would tour the grounds in his wheelchair. He would greet everyone kindly and warmly, never overstaying his welcome. One day he asked me why I was in the Palliative Care Ward and when I told him I had HIV, he nodded his head in sympathy. But the funny part to this story comes when I would see him again, he would ask, "so, how's your HIV?" It came as though he were asking how the gout was treating me? He was sincere, like many elderly people he didn't have much information about HIV, except that it was a disease, and that I was ill, just like he was ill. He was incorporating his knowledge with new knowledge, and he didn't look for the differences between us. Instead, he found the similarities; because he was a compassionate man.

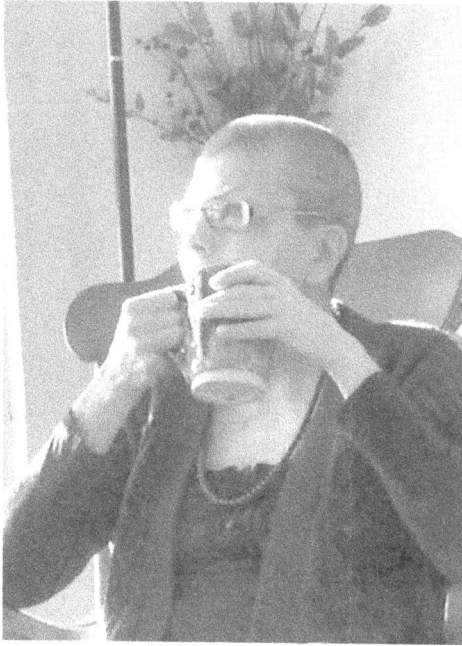

Gisele is a 53 year old widow with three adult children. She has a degree in Dramatic Studies and a Teaching Certificate. She taught English and French to middle and senior high students for 20 years.

"The first two words I wrote in a blog about two years ago were: . . . at last. After 25 years of living with HIV, I could speak the words, live the life I had let this virus take from me.

My husband died of AIDS in 1990. I carried on, keeping up with my children, my work and appearances. I have long been obsessed with poetry and have been published in numerous websites."

Dear Readers, all proceeds from the sales of this book will be donated to the charitable HIV/AIDS organization: The Stephen Lewis Foundation, established in March 2003. The organization provides support to grassroots projects. The sub-Saharan areas of Southern and Eastern Africa have been hit the hardest by the pandemic with some of the highest numbers of people living with HIV/AIDS.

The Foundation provides funding for initiatives for women with HIV/AIDS; offering social support, bereavement counselling, HIV testing and counselling, home and hospital care visits, and grants/loans for small income-generating projects to help women living with HIV/AIDS to support their families.

Stephen Lewis Foundation Grandmothers to grandmothers campaign seeks to raise awareness and mobilize support for African grandmothers struggling to provide a future for their grandchildren orphaned or made vulnerable due to HIV/AIDS. All proceeds from this book will be channelled to this campaign.

Lightning Source UK Ltd.
Milton Keynes UK
UKHW011445021120
372653UK00001B/345